2000 Calorie Diet

A Comprehensive Guide to Losing Weight and Keeping it Off

This book is a work of non-fiction. Any resemblance to actual people, places, or events is coincidental.

Published by Crown Publishers

Contents

Overview of Weight Loss Diet

When it comes to weight loss, a healthy diet is key. Eating a balanced diet that contains the right amounts of carbohydrates, proteins, and fats can help you lose weight and maintain your ideal weight. Below is an overview of what a weight loss diet should include.

Carbohydrates: Carbohydrates are an important source of energy and should make up 45-65 percent of your daily diet. Choose complex carbohydrates such as whole grains, fruits, and vegetables. These will give you a sustained energy boost and will help you feel fuller for longer.

Proteins: Proteins are essential for muscle growth and should make up 10-35 percent of your daily diet. Choose lean proteins such as fish, poultry, and eggs. These will help you feel full and will provide your body with essential amino acids.

Fats: Fats are an important part of a healthy diet and should make up 20-35 percent of your daily diet. Choose healthy fats such as olive oil, avocados, nuts, and seeds. These will help you feel full and provide your body with essential fatty acids.

In addition to eating the right foods, it is also important to watch your portion sizes. Eating too much can cause weight gain, so it is important to pay attention to how much you are eating.

Following a healthy weight loss diet will

help you reach your weight loss goals.

By eating the right foods and watching

your portion sizes, you will be well on

your way to achieving your ideal

weight.

Benefits of a Weight Loss Diet

A weight loss diet is a great way to achieve your weight loss goals. There are a variety of benefits to following a weight loss diet, including improved health, increased energy, and better body composition.

When you follow a weight loss diet, you will be consuming fewer calories than you would if you were eating a normal diet. This will result in healthier weight loss. You will also be able to reduce your risk of developing chronic diseases such as diabetes, high blood pressure, and heart disease.

A weight loss diet also provides you with more energy. When you reduce your calorie intake, your body will begin to use stored fat as a source of energy. This will help you to stay active and alert throughout the day.

Finally, a weight loss diet will help you to achieve a better body composition.

A healthy diet will help you to lose fat and build muscle. This will result in a leaner, healthier body.

Overall, a weight loss diet can provide you with a variety of benefits. It can help you to lose weight in a healthy way, increase your energy levels, and achieve a better body composition. A weight loss diet is an excellent way to reach your weight loss goals.

Goals of the Weight Loss Diet

When it comes to weight loss, it is important to have clear goals in mind. This will help you stay motivated and on track, so that you can reach your ultimate weight loss goals.

The first goal of any weight loss diet should be to create a caloric deficit. This means that you should be eating fewer calories than you are burning. You can do this by cutting out unhealthy foods from your diet and replacing them with healthier options.

The second goal of a weight loss diet should be to increase your intake of fiber. Fiber is important for helping to keep you feeling full and can also help to reduce your risk of developing certain diseases. You can increase your fiber intake by eating more vegetables, fruits, and whole grains.

The third goal of a weight loss diet should be to increase your intake of lean proteins. Lean proteins are important for helping to build and maintain muscle mass and can also help to keep you feeling full. You can increase your lean protein intake by eating more lean meats, fish, eggs, and beans.

Finally, the fourth goal of a weight loss diet should be to reduce your intake of added sugars and processed foods. These types of foods can lead to weight gain and are best avoided when trying to lose weight.

By following these goals, you will be well on your way to achieving your weight loss goals. Remember to keep your goals realistic and to reward yourself along the way. With dedication and perseverance, you will be able to reach your ultimate weight loss goals.

Establishing Your Goals for Weight Loss

When it comes to weight loss, it is important to have a plan and set realistic goals. This will help you stay motivated and on track, so that you can reach your ultimate weight loss goals.

The first step to establishing your goals is to determine what your ideal weight is. This will depend on your current body composition and your desired body composition. You can use a Body Mass Index (BMI) calculator to help you determine your ideal weight.

Once you know your ideal weight, you should set a goal for how much weight you would like to lose. You should also set a timeline for when you would like to reach your goal. It is important to keep your timeline realistic, so that you don't become discouraged if you don't meet your goal in the given timeframe.

In addition to setting a goal weight and timeline, you should also consider setting additional goals such as exercising regularly and eating healthier. These goals will help keep you motivated and on track with your weight loss plan.

You should also consider setting smaller goals along the way. These goals could be anything from eating a healthy breakfast every morning to going for a walk every evening. Setting smaller goals will give you something

to work towards and will help you stay
motivated.

Finally, it is important to reward
yourself for meeting your goals. This
will help keep you motivated and give
you something to look forward to as
you work towards your ultimate weight
loss goals.

By following these steps, you will be
well on your way to achieving your
weight loss goals. Remember to keep
your goals realistic and to reward

yourself along the way. With dedication and perseverance, you will be able to reach your ultimate weight loss goals.

Understanding Your Body

Your body is a complex and amazing machine. It is important to take the time to understand how your body works and how to take care of it. This will help you reach your health and fitness goals, and maintain your well-being.

The first step to understanding your body is to know your body types. There are three main body types: ectomorph, mesomorph, and endomorph. Ectomorphs are typically slender and have a difficult time gaining weight. Mesomorphs are typically muscular and athletic and can gain and lose weight easily. Endomorphs are typically rounder and have a harder time losing weight. Identifying your body type can help you better understand your body and the type of diet and exercise regimen that will work best for you.

The next step to understanding your body is to understand the different systems that make up your body. These include the muscular system, skeletal system, circulatory system, respiratory system, digestive system, and nervous system. Understanding how each of these systems works can help you better understand how your body works and how to take care of it.

Finally, it is important to understand how to recognize signs of illness or injury in your body. This includes being able to recognize the symptoms of common illnesses such as the flu, colds, and allergies, as well as signs of more serious conditions such as heart disease, cancer, and diabetes. Being able to recognize signs of illness or injury can help you take the necessary steps to get the help you need.

By taking the time to understand your body, you will be able to reach your health and fitness goals and maintain your well-being. Knowing your body type, understanding the different systems that make up your body, and recognizing signs of illness or injury can help you stay healthy and fit for

years to come.

Nutrition for Weight Loss

Good nutrition is an essential part of any successful weight loss program. Eating the right foods can help you lose weight, feel full, and provide your body with the necessary nutrients it needs to stay healthy.

The first step to creating a successful nutrition plan for weight loss is to identify your current eating habits. Are you eating a balanced diet that includes plenty of fruits and vegetables? Are you avoiding processed foods, sugars, and high-calorie beverages? Are you eating too much or too little? Identifying these habits will help you understand what changes you need to make in order to reach your weight loss goals.

Once you have identified your current eating habits, you should create a plan for how you will change your diet. Start by making small changes and gradually increasing the amount of fruits, vegetables, and whole grains in your diet. Additionally, you should reduce your intake of processed foods, sugars, and high-calorie beverages.

In addition to changing your diet, you should also focus on portion control. Eating smaller portions will help you reduce your overall calorie intake and will help you reach your weight loss goals.

Finally, it is important to stay hydrated. Drinking plenty of water throughout the day will help you feel full and will help you maintain your energy levels.

By following these steps, you will be well on your way to creating a successful nutrition plan for weight loss. Remember to make small changes and focus on portion control, and you will be able to reach your weight loss goals.

A 2,000-Calorie Diet: Food Lists and Meal Plan

Why 2,000 calories are often considered standard

Though nutritional requirements vary by individual, 2,000 calories are often considered standard.

This number is based on the estimated nutritional needs of most adults and used for meal-planning purposes according to the 2015–2020 Dietary Guidelines.

Additionally, it's used as a benchmark to create recommendations on nutrition labels.

In fact, all nutrition labels contain the phrase: "Percent Daily Values are based on a 2,000-calorie diet. Your Daily Values may be higher or lower depending on your calorie needs".

Due to these daily values, consumers can compare, for example, amounts of sodium and saturated fat in a given food to the maximum daily recommended levels.

Why calorie needs differ

Calories supply your body with the energy it needs to sustain life.

Because everyone's body and lifestyle is different, people have different calorie needs.

Depending on activity level, it's estimated that adult women require 1,600–2,400 calories per day, compared with 2,000–3,000 calories for adult men.

However, calorie needs vary drastically, with some people requiring more or fewer than 2,000 calories per day.

Additionally, individuals who are in periods of growth, such as pregnant women and teenagers, often need more than the standard 2,000 calories per day.

When the number of calories you burn is greater than the number you consume, a calorie deficit occurs, potentially resulting in weight loss.

Conversely, you may gain weight when you consume more calories than you burn. Weight maintenance occurs when both numbers are equal.

Therefore, depending on your weight goals and activity level, the appropriate number of calories you should consume differs.

Summary

The average adult needs approximately 2,000 calories per day. Yet, individual calorie recommendations depend on many factors, such as your size, gender, exercise level, weight goals, and overall health.

Exercise for Weight Loss

Exercise is an important part of any weight loss plan. Regular exercise can help you burn calories, build muscle, and increase your overall health and well-being. When it comes to weight loss, it is important to choose the right type of exercise and to do it regularly.

The best type of exercise for weight loss is aerobic exercise. This includes activities such as running, walking, biking, swimming, and other activities that get your heart rate up and make you sweat. Aim to do at least 30 minutes of aerobic exercise 3-5 days a week.

Strength training is also beneficial for weight loss. Strength training helps build muscle, which can help you burn more calories. Aim to do strength training at least twice a week.

In addition to aerobic and strength training, it is also important to do stretching and flexibility exercises.

This will help keep you flexible and reduce the risk of injury. Try to do at least 10 minutes of stretching and flexibility exercises every day.

Finally, it is important to find activities that you enjoy. Exercise should be something that you look forward to and that you will stick with in the long run. Don't be afraid to try new activities or vary your routine.

By following these tips, you will be well on your way to achieving your weight loss goals. Remember to be consistent, find activities that you enjoy, and be patient. With dedication and perseverance, you will be able to reach your ultimate weight loss goals.

Can a 2,000-calorie diet aid weight loss?

Following a 2,000-calorie diet may help some people lose weight. Its effectiveness for this purpose depends on your age, gender, height, weight, activity level, and weight loss goals.

It's important to note that weight loss is much more complicated than simply reducing your calorie intake. Other factors that affect weight loss include your environment, socioeconomic factors, and even your gut bacteria.

That said, calorie restriction is one of the main targets in obesity prevention and management.

For example, if you reduce your daily calorie intake from 2,500 to 2,000, you should lose 1 pound (0.45 kg) in 1 week, as 3,500 calories (500 calories saved over 7 days) is the approximate number of calories in 1 pound of body fat.

On the other hand, a 2,000-calorie diet would exceed the calorie needs of some people, likely resulting in weight gain.

Summary

Though 2,000-calorie diets have the potential to aid weight loss, it's important to tailor your intake to your individual needs, as calorie needs vary based on many factors.

Foods to eat

A well-balanced, healthy diet includes plenty of whole, unprocessed foods.

Where your calories come from is just as important as how many calories you consume.

While it's vital to ensure that you're getting enough carbs, protein, and fat, a focus on foods rather than macronutrients may be more helpful to create a healthy diet.

At each meal, you should focus on high-quality protein and fiber-rich foods, such as fruits, vegetables, and whole grains.

While you can indulge on occasion, your diet should mainly consist of the following types of foods:

- Whole grains: brown rice, oats, bulgur, quinoa, farro, millet, etc.

- Fruits: berries, peaches, apples, pears, melons, bananas, grapes, etc.

- Non-starchy vegetables: kale, spinach, peppers, zucchini, broccoli, bok choy, Swiss chard, tomatoes, cauliflower, etc.

- Starchy vegetables: butternut squash, sweet potatoes, winter squash, potatoes, peas, plantains, etc.

- Dairy products: reduced or full-fat plain yogurt, kefir, and full-fat cheeses.

- Lean meats: turkey, chicken, beef, lamb, bison, veal, etc.

- Nuts, nut butters, and seeds: almonds, cashews, macadamia nuts, hazelnuts, sunflower seeds, pine nuts, and natural nut butters

- Fish and seafood: tuna, salmon, halibut, scallops, mussels, clams, shrimp, etc.

- Legumes: chickpeas, black beans, cannellini beans, kidney beans, lentils, etc.

- Eggs: organic, whole eggs are the healthiest and most nutrient dense

- Plant-based protein: tofu, edamame, tempeh, seitan, plant-based protein powders, etc.

- Healthy fats: avocados, coconut oil, avocado oil, olive oil, etc.

- Spices: ginger, turmeric, black pepper, red pepper, paprika, cinnamon, nutmeg, etc.

- Herbs: parsley, basil, dill, cilantro, oregano, rosemary, tarragon, etc.

- Calorie-free beverages: black coffee, tea, sparkling water, etc.

Studies suggest that adding a protein source to meals and snacks can help promote feelings of fullness and aid weight loss and maintenance.

Additionally, monitoring your carb intake and choosing the right types of carbs can assist with weight maintenance.

It's important to eat a variety of whole, unprocessed foods — not only to meet your nutritional needs but also to achieve and maintain a healthy weight and promote optimal health.

Summary

A balanced, healthy diet should consist of a variety of whole, unprocessed foods, including plenty of fruits, vegetables, lean protein, legumes, whole grains, and healthy fats.

Foods to avoid

It's best to avoid foods that provide little to no nutritional value — also known as "empty calories." These are

typically foods that are high in calories
and added sugars yet low in nutrients.

Here is a list of foods to avoid or limit
on any healthy diet, regardless of your
calorie needs:

• Added sugars: agave, baked goods,
ice cream, candy, etc. — limit added
sugars to less than 5–10% of your
total calories

• Fast food: French fries, hot dogs,
pizza, chicken nuggets, etc.

• Processed and refined carbs: bagels,
white bread, crackers, cookies, chips,
sugary cereals, boxed pasta, etc.

- Fried foods: French fries, fried chicken, doughnuts, potato chips, fish and chips, etc.

- Sodas and sugar-sweetened beverages: sports drinks, sugary juices, sodas, fruit punch, sweetened tea and coffee drinks, etc.

- Diet and low-fat foods: diet ice cream, diet boxed snacks, diet packaged and frozen meals, and artificial sweeteners, such as Sweet n' Low, etc.

Though most of your diet should consist of whole, unprocessed foods, it's okay to indulge in less healthy foods occasionally.

However, regularly eating the foods on this list may not only be harmful to your health but also delay or hinder weight loss or even disrupt your weight maintenance efforts.

Summary

It's best to avoid or limit foods with little to no nutritional value, such as fried foods, refined carbs, and sugary snacks and beverages.

Sample meal plan

Here's a healthy 5-day sample meal plan with approximately 2,000 calories per day.

Each meal contains approximately 500 calories and each snack about 250 calories.

Monday

Breakfast: vegetable omelet

- 2 eggs

- 1 cup (20 grams) of spinach

- 1/4 cup (24 grams) of mushrooms

- 1/4 cup (23 grams) of broccoli

- 1 cup (205 grams) of sautéed sweet potatoes

- 1 tablespoon (15 ml) of olive oil

Snack: apple with peanut butter

- 1 medium apple

- 2 tablespoons (32 grams) of peanut butter

Lunch: Mediterranean tuna pita pockets

- 1 whole-wheat pita

- 5 ounces (140 grams) of canned tuna

- chopped red onion and celery

- 1/4 avocado

- 1 tablespoon (9 grams) of crumbled feta cheese

Snack: cheese and grapes

- 2 ounces (56 grams) of cheddar cheese

- 1 cup (92 grams) of grapes

Dinner: salmon with veggies and wild rice

- 5 ounces (140 grams) of baked salmon

* 2 tablespoons (30 ml) of olive oil

* 1/2 cup (82 grams) of cooked wild rice

* 1 cup (180 grams) of roasted asparagus

* 1 cup (100 grams) of roasted eggplant

Tuesday

Breakfast: nut butter and banana toast

* 2 slices of whole-grain toast

* 2 tablespoons (32 grams) of almond butter

- 1 sliced banana

- cinnamon to sprinkle on top

Snack: power smoothie

- 3/4 cup (180 ml) of unsweetened, non-dairy milk

- 1 cup (20 grams) of spinach

- 1 scoop (42 grams) of plant-based protein powder

- 1 cup (123 grams) of frozen blueberries

- 1 tablespoon (14 grams) of hemp seeds

Lunch: avocado-tuna salad

- 1/2 avocado

- 5 ounces (140 grams) of canned tuna

- 1/2 cup (75 grams) of cherry tomatoes

- 2 cups (100–140 grams) of mixed greens

Lunch: black bean and sweet potato burrito

- 1 whole-wheat tortilla

- 1/4 cup (41 grams) of cooked brown rice

- 1/2 cup (102 grams) of cooked sweet potatoes

- 1/4 cup (50 grams) of black beans

- 2 tablespoons (30 grams) of salsa

Snack: vegetables and hummus

- fresh carrot and celery sticks

- 2 tablespoons (30 grams) of hummus

- 1/2 whole-wheat pita bread

Dinner: chicken and broccoli stir-fry

- 5 ounces (140 grams) of chicken

- 2 cups (176 grams) of broccoli

- 1/2 cup (82 grams) of cooked brown rice

- fresh garlic and ginger

- 1 tablespoon (15 ml) of soy sauce

Wednesday

Breakfast: berry yogurt parfait

- 7 ounces (200 grams) of plain Greek yogurt

- 1/2 cup (74 grams) of fresh blueberries

- 1/2 cup (76 grams) of sliced strawberries

- 1/4 cup (30 grams) of granola

Snack: banana and almond butter

- 1 banana

- 1 1/2 tablespoons (24 grams) of almond butter

Lunch: peanut noodles with tofu and peas

- 3/4 cup (132 grams) of cooked rice noodles

- 5 ounces (141 grams) of tofu

- 1/2 cup (125 grams) of peas

- 1 tablespoon (16 grams) of creamy peanut butter

- 2 teaspoons (10 grams) of tamari or soy sauce

- 1/2 teaspoon (2 grams) of Sriracha

- 2 teaspoons (14 grams) of honey

- juice of 1/2 lime

Snack: protein bar

- Look for bars containing approximately 200–250 calories with less than 12 grams of sugar and at least 5 grams of fiber.

Dinner: fish tacos

* 3 corn tortillas

* 6 ounces (170 grams) of grilled cod

* 1/2 avocado

* 2 tablespoons (34 grams) of pico de
gallo

Thursday

Breakfast: avocado toast with egg

* 1/2 avocado

* 2 slices of whole-wheat toast

* 1 tablespoon (15 ml) of olive oil

* 1 egg

Snack: Greek yogurt with strawberries

• 7 ounces (200 grams) of plain Greek yogurt

• 3/4 cup (125 grams) of sliced strawberries

Lunch: quinoa with mixed vegetables and grilled chicken

• 1/2 cup (93 grams) of cooked quinoa

• 5 ounces (142 grams) of grilled chicken

• 1 tablespoon (15 ml) of olive oil

• 1 cup (180 grams) of mixed, non-starchy vegetables

Snack: dark chocolate and almonds

- 2 squares (21 grams) of dark chocolate

- 15–20 almonds

Dinner: vegetarian chili

- 1/2 cup (121 grams) of canned, crushed tomatoes

- 1/2 cup (130 grams) of kidney beans

- 1/2 cup (103 grams) of butternut squash

- 1/2 cup (75 grams) of cooked sweet corn

- 1/4 cup (28 grams) of diced white onions

- 1/4 of a jalapeño pepper

Friday

Breakfast: oatmeal with seeds and dried fruit

- 1/2 cups (80 grams) of steel-cut oats

- 1 tablespoon (14 grams) of hemp seeds

- 1 tablespoon (12 grams) of flax seeds

- 2 tablespoons (20 grams) of dried cherries

Snack: bell peppers and carrots with guacamole

- 1/2 bell pepper, cut into strips

- 1 cup of carrot sticks

- 4 tablespoons (60 grams) of guacamole

Lunch: grilled vegetable and mozzarella wrap

- 1 whole-wheat tortilla

- 1/2 cup (60 grams) of grilled red peppers

- 5 slices (42 grams) of grilled zucchini

- 3 ounces (84 grams) of fresh mozzarella

Snack: chia pudding with banana

- 5 ounces (170 grams) of chia pudding

- 1/2 of a sliced banana

Dinner: pasta with pesto, peas, and shrimp

- 2 tablespoons (30 grams) of pesto

- 1/2 cup (42 grams) of whole-wheat or brown-rice penne

- 6 ounces (170 grams) of shrimp

- 1/2 cup (80 grams) of peas

- 1 tablespoon (5 grams) of grated Parmesan cheese

A healthy and well-balanced diet can be both delicious and nourishing. This 2,000-calorie sample menu consists of meals with whole, unprocessed foods. Plus, it's rich in fiber, protein, fruit, vegetables, and healthy fats.

With a little planning and preparation, achieving a nutritious diet can be easy. Also, it's possible to find similar meals similar when dining out.

Nevertheless, it's often easier to make healthier choices and control portion sizes when you prepare your meals at home from fresh ingredients.

Summary

A 2,000-calorie diet should consist of whole, unprocessed foods and be rich in fruits, vegetables, protein, whole grains, and healthy fats. Planning and preparing your meals makes it easier to eat a healthy, balanced diet.

The bottom line

A 2,000-calorie diet meets the needs of most adults.

Still, individual needs vary depending on your age, gender, weight, height, activity level, and weight goals.

As with any healthy diet, a 2,000-calorie diet should include whole, unprocessed foods like fresh produce, protein, and healthy fats.

2,000-Calorie Diets for Men

Healthy man.

Although 2,000-calorie diets often lead to weight loss in men, some men do require 2,000 calories a day to maintain a healthy body weight. The number of calories a man should consume daily depends on his age, his size, his activity level and his weight-management goals. Following a daily 2,000-calorie meal plan will likely help you achieve your weight-loss goals.

According to the Dietary Guidelines for Americans 2010, sedentary men over age 60 often need 2,000 calories daily to maintain a healthy body weight. However, sedentary men and moderately active men 60 and younger need at least 2,200 calories a day for healthy weight maintenance. Active men ages 19 to 35 need as many as 3,000 calories a day to maintain their body weight. Therefore, many men who consume 2,000 calories a day will start to lose weight.

If a 2,000-calorie diet is appropriate for you, using a meal plan will help you stay within your daily allowance of calories. According to the 2010 Dietary Guidelines, a daily 2,000-calorie healthy meal plan includes 6 ounces of grains, 5.5 ounces of protein foods, 3 cups of dairy foods, 6 teaspoons of oils, 2.5 cups of vegetables, 2 cups of fruits and 258 extra calories from foods that you choose. Select whole grains when possible, and avoid sweets, added sugars and high-fat meats.

Sample Menu 1

Grilled chicken and rice.

For breakfast, try two slices of whole-grain toast, 1 tablespoon of peanut butter, four egg whites, one small orange and 1 cup of low-fat Greek yogurt. A mid-morning snack might consist of 1.5 ounces of reduced-fat cheese and 1 cup of blueberries. For lunch, opt for 2.5 ounces of grilled chicken breast, 1 cup of brown rice and 1.25 cups of cooked broccoli. A good choice for a healthy afternoon snack is two-thirds of an ounce of sunflower seeds and 2 cups of low-fat cottage cheese. For dinner, have 2.5 ounces of cooked lean beef; 1.25 cups of sautéed mushrooms, onions and peppers; 2 teaspoons of olive oil; and 1 cup of whole-wheat pasta.

Sample Menu 2

Whole grain cereal and a banana.

Start your day with a healthy breakfast of 2 cups of whole-grain cereal, 1.5 cups of low-fat milk, one small banana and two-thirds of an ounce of almonds. For a morning snack, opt for 1 cup of low-fat cottage cheese and 1 cup of strawberries. A healthy lunch might consist of 3 ounces of grilled salmon, 1 cup of quinoa and 1.5 cups of cooked zucchini. For an afternoon snack, have two-thirds of an ounce of mixed nuts and 1 cup of low-fat yogurt. A healthy dinner could include a turkey burger on a whole-grain bun, 2 cups of mixed greens and 2 tablespoons of Italian

salad dressing.